I0113417

Vegetarian Diet Cookbook

A Fresh Guide To Eating Well With Delicious Recipes For A Healthy Balanced Diet

Brigitte S. Romeo

© Copyright 2021 - All rights reserved.

The content contained within this book may not be reproduced, duplicated or transmitted without direct written permission from the author or the publisher.

Under no circumstances will any blame or legal responsibility be held against the publisher, or author, for any damages, reparation, or monetary loss due to the information contained within this book. Either directly or indirectly.

Legal Notice:

This book is copyright protected. This book is only for personal use. You cannot amend, distribute, sell, use, quote or paraphrase any part, or the content within this book, without the consent of the author or publisher.

Disclaimer Notice:

Please note the information contained within this document is for educational and entertainment purposes only. All effort has been executed to present accurate, up to date, and reliable, complete information. No warranties of any kind are declared or implied. Readers acknowledge that the author is not engaging in the rendering of legal, financial, medical or professional advice. The content within this book has been derived from various sources. Please consult a licensed professional before attempting any techniques outlined in this book.

By reading this document, the reader agrees that under no circumstances is the author responsible for any losses, direct or indirect, which are incurred as a result of the use of information contained within this document, including, but not limited to, errors, omissions, or inaccuracies.

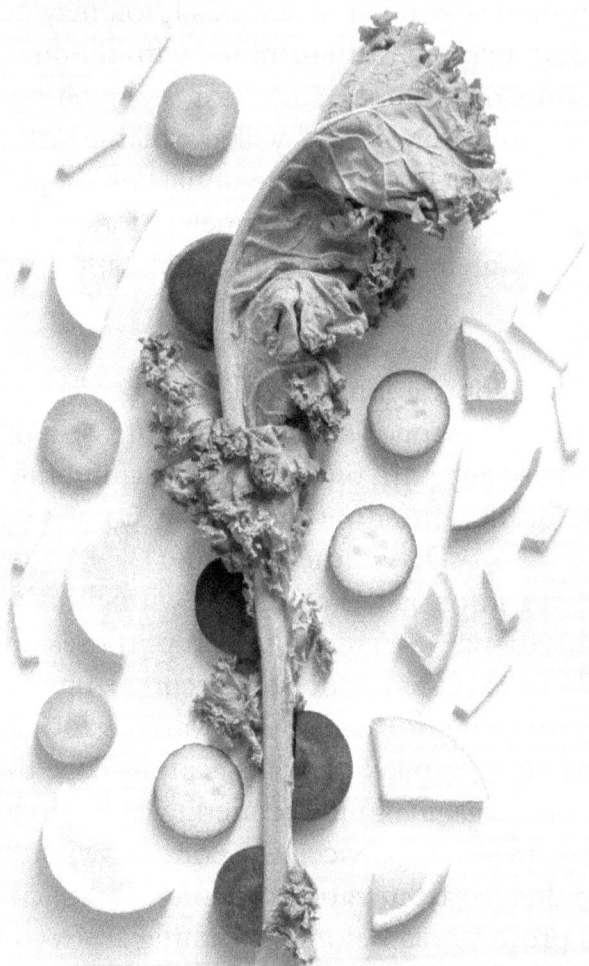

TABLE OF CONTENTS

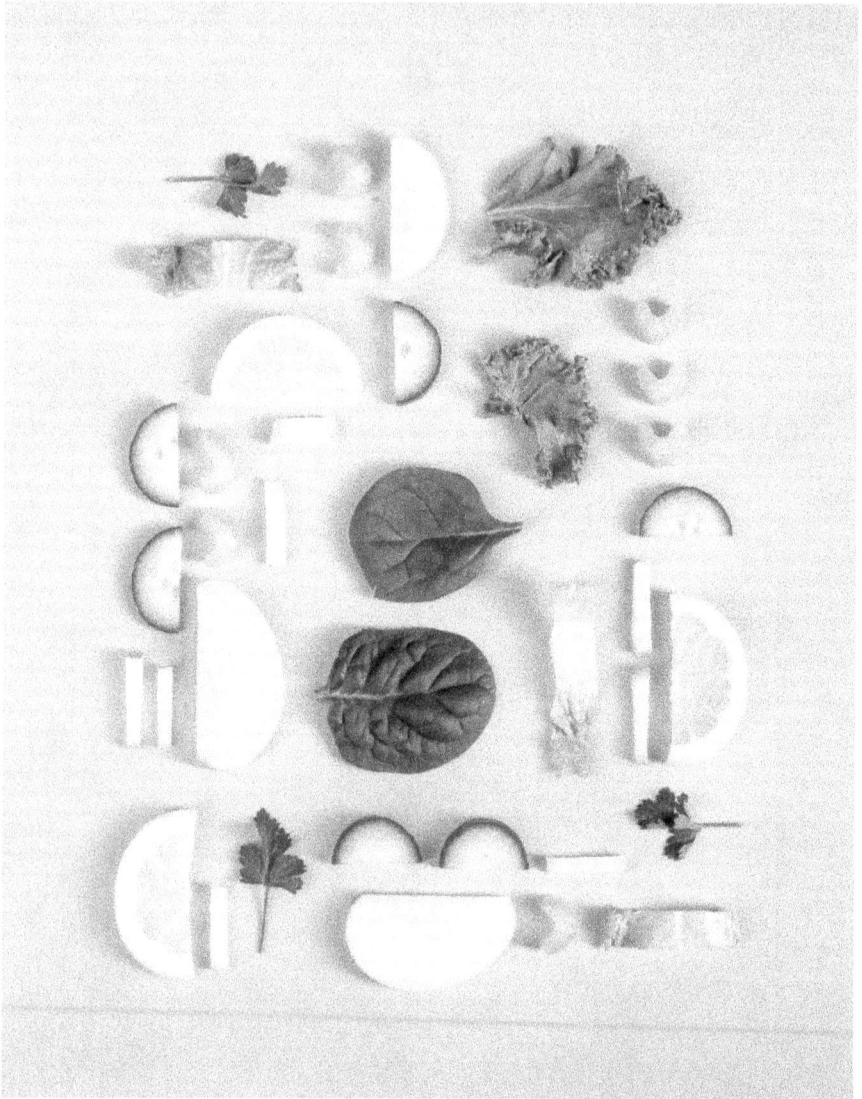

INTRODUCTION

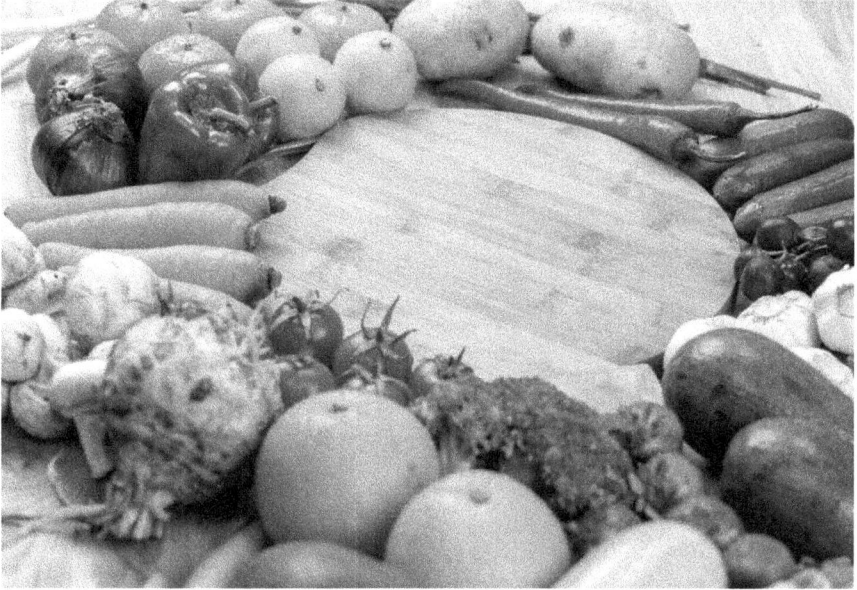

What does it mean to be a vegetarian?

A Vegetarian is a person who does not eat meat, poultry, or fish. Vegetarians eat only plant foods such as fruits, vegetables, legumes, and grains or products made from them. Some people think of a vegetarian as a person who does not eat red meat but may consume fish and chicken. Other people consider a vegetarian to be someone who avoids eating all animal flesh, including fish, poultry, and red meat. However, "true" vegetarians avoid the consumption of all meats, including fish and chicken.

How often should you eat fruits and vegetables? The recommendation is to eat five servings per day based on a 2,000 calorie diet. One serving is equal to one-half cup raw or one cup ready-to-eat. Fruits and vegetables provide vitamins, minerals, fiber, and other nutrients that are essential for good health. It is recommended that most Americans make fruits and vegetables the basis of their diet; ideally, they should be eaten at every meal.

So, specifically, what are the foods that one needs to avoid? These are as follows:

- Beef

- Pork

- Lamb

- Veal

- All Game (deer, elk, etc.)

- Any other land mammal that's been fed animal products or by-products such as eggs and dairy (many land mammals are herbivores)

- Fish and Shellfish

- Goose and Duck

- Emu and Alligator

- Any other animal that is not a seafood product

- Animal by-products such as gelatin (e.g., gummy bears)

As a vegetarian, what specific foods do you avoid? For starters, you can limit your consumption of the following:

- Pork and bacon

- Eggs (or eat only eggs that are certified organic or non-cage free)

- Dairy products (or consume only dairy products that are certified organic)

- All products that are made from animals, such as leather shoes, belts, jackets, etc.

What are the substitutes that you use to replace the meat and fish that you avoid?

- Tofu (made from soybeans)

- Tempeh (made from soybeans)

- TVP (textured vegetable protein)

- Seitan (very high in protein, available as steak strips or chicken-style pieces)

- Soy Nuggets/Sausage

Being a vegetarian has its benefits, but there are definitely some challenges as well. If you are considering the option of being a vegetarian, the most important thing to consider is your overall health. However, if you have concerns with the lack of protein in your diet, believe that it's unwise to eat only plant products, or simply crave meat and fish and think you can't give them up without feeling hungry or deprived, then the choice of becoming a vegetarian may not be the right one for you.

This vegetarian cookbook will help you get a delicious and healthy recipe on the table that will make your life less stressful. A good recipe doesn't need a long list of ingredients to make it tasty, and while preparing meals may seem hard. You can eat together a healthy family food in the same amount of time you'd need to order takeout!

This vegetarian cookbook will show you a variety of dishes you can make with easy-to-find ingredients. This is the perfect practical guide for anyone looking to make a variety of delicious meals that are healthy. It includes recipes for breakfast, lunch, dinner, appetizers, and desserts, as well as those for snacks and sides.

Whether looking to lose weight or just eat more healthily, this cookbook will make it easier than ever before!

So, let us begin the journey.

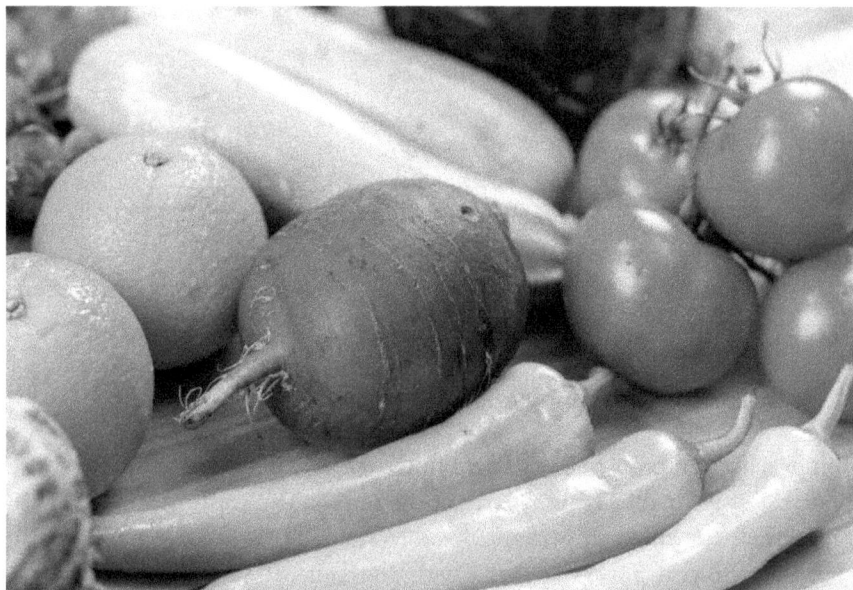

CHAPTER 1:

BREAKFAST RECIPES

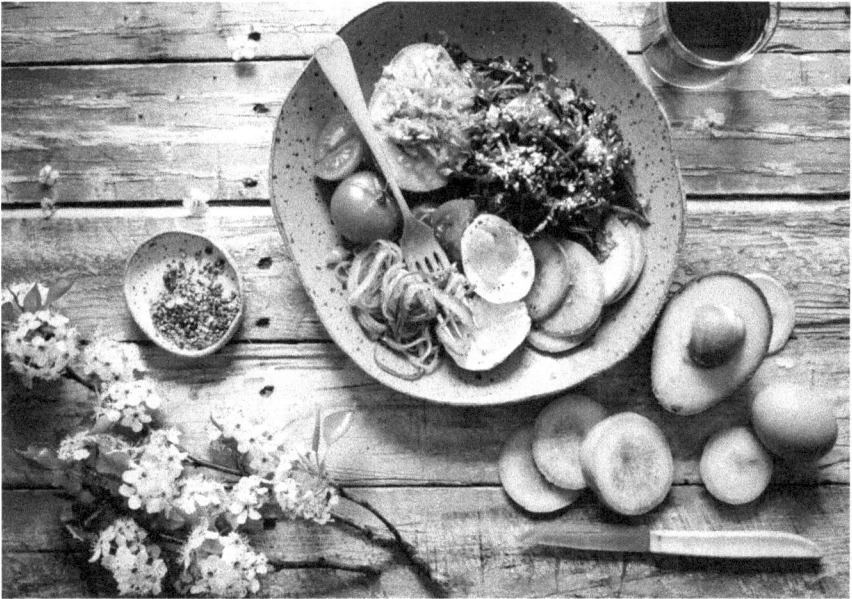

1. Overnight Chia Seed Plant-Powered Breakfast

Preparation Time: 5 minutes

Cooking Time: 0 minutes

Servings: 3

Ingredients:

- ½ cup chia seeds

- 2 cups unsweetened almond milk or any unflavored, unsweetened non-dairy milk

- 3 tablespoons pure maple syrup

- ½ teaspoon vanilla extract

- Toppings of your choice: fruits, nuts, seeds, figs, dates, toasted coconut flakes (optional)

Directions:

1. In a container with a lid, thoroughly combine the chia seeds, almond milk, maple syrup, and vanilla. Refrigerate overnight until it becomes thick and pudding-like.

2. When you're ready to serve, stir to remove any clumps. Spoon into bowls and customize your breakfast by adding your favorite toppings. I like to include a sweet and crunchy element. Drizzle with a little extra maple syrup, if you'd like.

Nutrition: Calories: 397 Fat: 21g Carbohydrate: 46g Protein: 10g

2. <u>Baked Oatmeal and Fruit</u>

Preparation Time: 5 minutes

Cooking Time: 20 minutes

Servings: 4

Ingredients:

- 3 cups quick-cooking oats

- 3 cups unflavored, unsweetened nondairy milk

- ¼ cup pure maple syrup

- 1 tablespoon vanilla extract

- 1 to 2 cups blueberries, raspberries, or both

Directions:

1. Preheat the oven to 375°F.

2. In a large mixing bowl, combine all the ingredients. Put everything in a large bowl, then cover it with aluminum foil.

3. Bake for 10 minutes, then bake for another 5 to 10 minutes uncovered, or until all the liquid is visibly gone and the edges start to brown.

4. Let cool 5 minutes before serving. Serve with an extra splash of non-dairy milk and a drizzle of maple syrup.

5. Leftovers: Make a big batch as a quick go-to breakfast for the week. Just reheat in the oven or microwave or on the stovetop.

Nutrition: Calories: 365 Fat: 7g Carbohydrate: 67g Protein: 9g

3. <u>Hemp and Oat Granola</u>

Preparation Time: 5 minutes

Cooking Time: 30 minutes

Servings: 4

Ingredients:

- 2 cups old-fashioned rolled oats

- 1½ teaspoons cinnamon

- ½ cup hemp seeds

- ⅓ Cup slivered almonds

- ⅓ Cup pure maple syrup

Directions:

1. Preheat the oven to 350°F. Line large baking sheet using parchment paper.

2. Spread the oats on the lined baking sheet. Sprinkle over the cinnamon and toss. Spread evenly on the baking sheet and toast in the oven for 10 minutes.

3. Add the hemp seeds and toss them with the oats. Toast for another 10 minutes. Add the almonds, toss, and toast for another 5 minutes.

4. Take it off the oven and drizzle with maple syrup. Toss, spread evenly on the baking sheet, and toast for another 5 minutes.

5. Refrigerate covered for up to 5 days.

6. Substitution Tip: Substitute sunflower seeds for the hemp seeds or add ½ cup chopped dates or dried fruit.

Nutrition: Calories: 434 Fat: 20g Carbohydrate: 49g Protein: 17g

4. <u>Quick Green Posole</u>

Preparation Time: 10 minutes

Cooking Time: 3 minutes

Servings: 4

Ingredients:

- 6 ounces (about 5) tomatillos, hulled, washed, and quartered

- ½ jalapeño, seeded and ribs removed, roughly chopped

- 1 small yellow onion, roughly chopped

- 2 (15-ounce) cans hominy, drained

- 1 cup vegetable broth

- 1 teaspoon ground cumin

- ½ teaspoon chili powder

- 1 teaspoon garlic powder

- ½ teaspoon dried oregano

- ¼ teaspoon kosher salt, plus more for seasoning

Directions:

1. Put the tomatillos, jalapeño, and onion in a blender and pulse to chop all the ingredients into a chunky purée. Pour mixture into the pressure cooker pot. Add the hominy, vegetable broth, cumin, chili powder, garlic powder, oregano, and salt.

2. Lock the pressure cooker and then set the timer for 3 minutes at low pressure. When the timer is off, quick release the pressure. Stir the mixture to recombine, add additional salt if needed, and serve immediately.

Nutrition: Calories: 289 Carbs: 37g Fat: 10g Protein: 16g

5. <u>Harvest Ratatouille</u>

Preparation Time: 15 minutes

Cooking Time: 3 minutes

Servings: 4

Ingredients:

- 2 tablespoons extra-virgin olive oil, divided

- 2 large yellow onions, diced

- 1 teaspoon garlic powder

- 1 teaspoon dried thyme

- 1 teaspoon dried oregano

- ½ teaspoon kosher salt, plus more if needed

- 1 eggplant, cut into 1-inch chunks

- 2 red bell peppers, seeded and diced

- 2 summer squash, sliced

- 1 (28-ounce) can whole tomatoes, in juice

- ¼ teaspoon freshly ground black pepper

Directions:

1. With the pressure cooker on the brown or sauté setting, heat 1 tablespoon of olive oil until it shimmers. Add the onions and sauté, stirring frequently, until they are softened and translucent, about 5 minutes. Stir in the garlic powder, thyme, oregano, and salt. Add the eggplant, bell peppers, and squash, and pour the tomatoes and their juices over the vegetables without stirring.

2. Lock the lid, then set the timer for 3 minutes at high pressure. When the timer is off, quick release the pressure. Gently stir the ingredients, drizzling in the remaining 1 tablespoon of olive oil, and season it with salt and pepper if needed. Serve hot or warm.

Nutrition: Calories: 189 Carbs: 15g Fat: 12g Protein: 3g

6. <u>Green Thai Tofu and Veggie Curry</u>

Preparation Time: 15 minutes

Cooking Time: 3 minutes

Servings: 4

Ingredients:

- 1 (14-ounce) block extra-firm tofu

- 2 red bell peppers, seeded and sliced

- 1 red onion, sliced

- 8 ounces green beans, trimmed into 1-inch

- 1 (14-ounce) can prepare green curry

Directions:

1. Slice the tofu lengthwise, then cut each piece into 1-inch cubes. Add the tofu, peppers, onion, and green beans to the pressure cooker pot. Pour curry sauce over the tofu and vegetables and stir lightly to combine.

2. Lock lid and set the timer for 3 minutes at high pressure. When the timer is off, quickly release the pressure. Stir to combine and serve immediately.

Nutrition: Calories: 170 Carbs: 8g Fat: 14g Protein: 6g

7. <u>Indian Chickpea Curry</u>

Preparation Time: 10 minutes

Cooking Time: 3 minutes

Servings: 4

Ingredients:

- 1 tablespoon vegetable oil

- 1 medium yellow onion, sliced

- 2 tablespoons red curry paste

- 1 (13.5-ounce) can coconut milk

- 2 teaspoons cornstarch

- 2 cups canned chickpeas or 2 cups Basic Chickpeas

- 4 carrots, peeled and sliced

Directions:

1. With the pressure cooker on the brown or sauté setting, heat the vegetable oil until it shimmers. Sauté the onion and stir frequently, until it is softened and translucent, about 5 minutes.

Stir in the curry paste and sauté, stirring constantly, for 1 minute. Stir in the coconut milk.

2. Place the cornstarch in a small bowl. Add a spoonful or two of warm liquid from the pot to the bowl and use a fork or spoon to make a loose paste. Stir cornstarch mixture back into the pot. Then add the chickpeas and carrots to the pot.

3. Lock lid and set the timer for 3 minutes at high pressure. When the timer is off, quickly release the pressure. Stir the curry and serve hot.

Nutrition: Calories: 332 Carbs: 55g Fat: 8g Protein: 10g

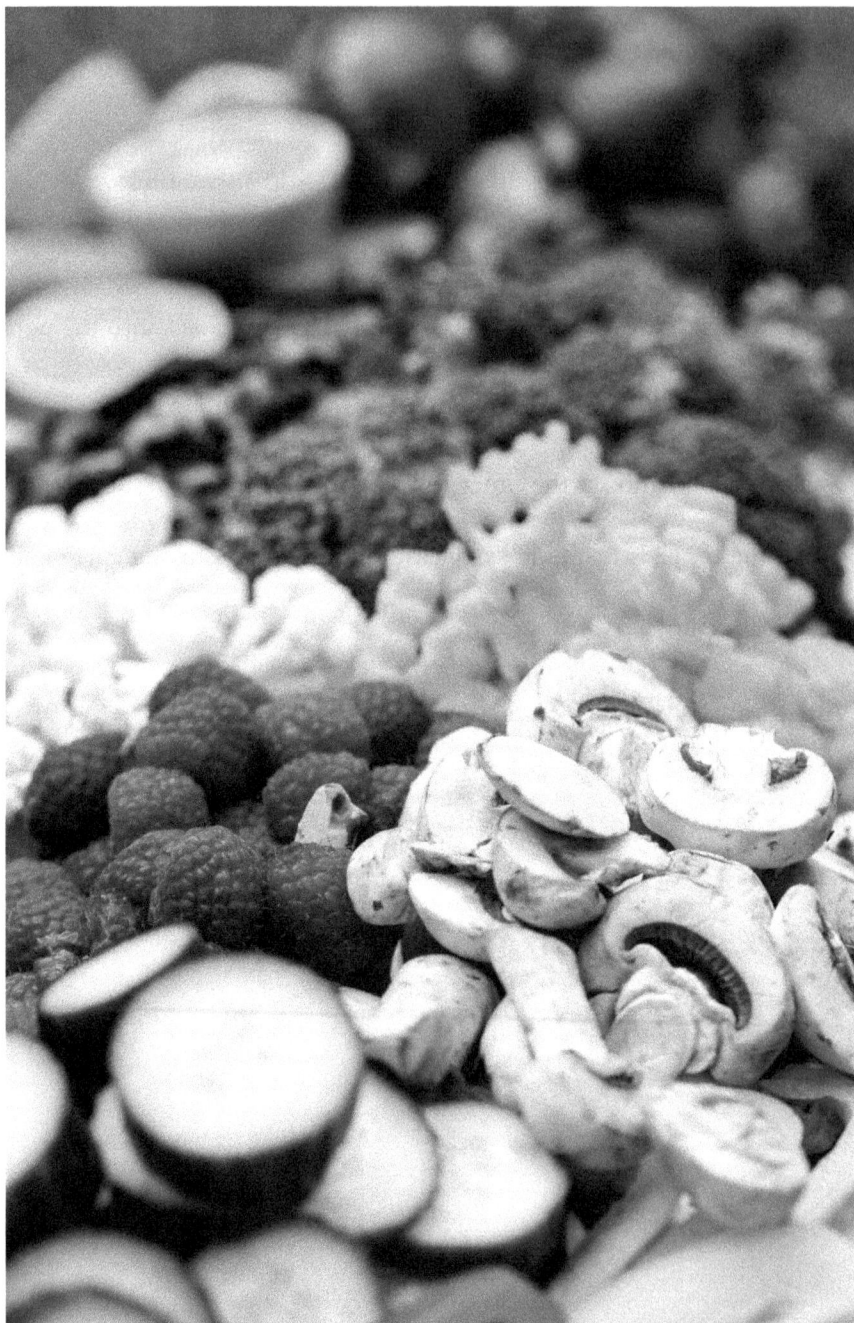

CHAPTER 2:

LUNCH RECIPES

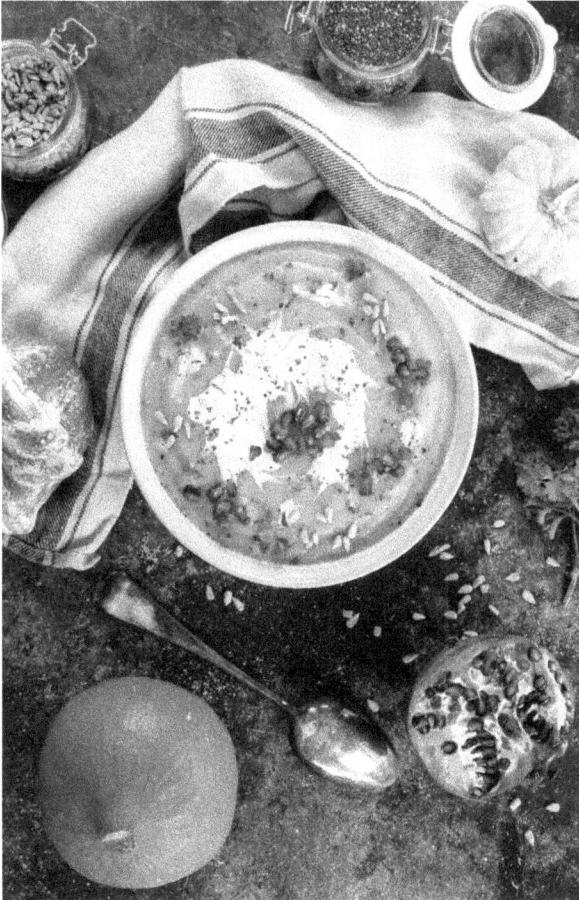

8. <u>Baked Mac and Peas</u>

Preparation Time: 15 minutes Cooking Time: 40 minutes

Servings: 8

Ingredients:

- 1 (16-ounce) package whole-wheat macaroni pasta

- 1 recipe Anytime "Cheese" Sauce

- 2 cups green peas (fresh or frozen)

Directions:

1. Preheat the oven to 400°F.

2. In a large stockpot, cook the pasta per the package instructions for al dente. Drain the pasta.

3. Combine the pasta, sauce, and peas, and mix well in a large baking dish.

4. Bake for 30 minutes, or until the top of the dish turns golden brown.

Nutrition: Calories: 209 Total fat: 3g Carbohydrates: 42g Fiber: 7g Protein: 12g

9. <u>Savory Sweet Potato Casserole</u>

Preparation Time: 15 minutes Cooking Time: 30 minutes

Servings: 6

Ingredients:

- 8 sweet potatoes, cooked

- ½ cup vegetable broth

- 1 tablespoon dried sage

- 1 teaspoon dried thyme

- 1 teaspoon dried rosemary

Directions:

1. Preheat the oven to 375°F.Peel the cooked sweet potatoes and put them in a baking dish. Mash sweet potatoes using a fork or potato masher. Then mix it in the broth, sage, thyme, and rosemary.

2. Bake for 30 minutes and serve.

Nutrition: Calories: 154 Total fat: 0g Carbohydrates: 35g Fiber: 6g Protein: 3g

10. White Bean and Chickpea Hummus

Preparation Time: 5 minutes

Cooking Time: 30 minutes

Servings: 8

Ingredients:

- 1 (15-ounce) can chickpeas

- 1 (15-ounce) can white beans (cannellini or great northern)

- 3 tablespoons freshly squeezed lemon juice

- 2 teaspoons garlic powder

- 1 teaspoon onion powder

Directions:

1. Prepare the chickpeas and white beans. Make sure to drain and rinse.

2. In a food processor or blender, combine the chickpeas, beans, lemon juice, garlic powder, and onion powder. Process for 1 to 2 minutes, or until the texture is smooth and creamy.

3. Serve right away, or store in a refrigerator-safe container for up to 5 days.

Nutrition: Calories: 69 Total fat: 1g Carbohydrates: 12g Fiber: 4g Protein: 4g

11. <u>Pesto Pearled Barley</u>

Preparation Time: 2 minutes

Cooking Time: 50 minutes

Servings: 4

Ingredients:

- 1 cup dried barley

- 2½ cups vegetable broth

- ½ cup Parm-y Kale Pesto

Directions:

1. In a medium saucepan, combine the barley and broth and bring to a boil. Cover, reduce the heat to low, and simmer for about 45 minutes, until tender. Remove from the stove and let stand for 5 minutes.

2. Fluff the barley, then gently fold in the pesto.

3. Scoop about ¾ cup into each of 4 single-compartment storage containers. Let cool before sealing the lids.

Nutrition: Calories: 237 Total fat: 6g Carbohydrates: 40g Fiber: 11g

12. Five-Spice Farro

Preparation Time: 3 minutes

Cooking Time: 35 minutes

Servings: 4

Ingredients:

- 1 cup dried faro, rinsed and drained

- 1 teaspoon five-spice powder

Directions:

1. In a medium pot, combine the farro, five-spice powder, and enough water to cover. Bring to a boil; reduce the heat to medium-low, and simmer for 30 minutes. Drain off any excess water.

2. Transfer to a large storage container, or scoop 1 cup farro into each of 4 storage containers. Let cool before sealing the lids.

Nutrition: Calories: 73 Total fat: 0g Carbohydrates: 15g Fiber: 1g

13. <u>Sushi-Style Quinoa</u>

Preparation Time: 2 minutes

Cooking Time: 25 minutes

Servings: 4

Ingredients:

- 2 cups water

- 1 cup dry quinoa, rinsed

- ¼ cup unseasoned rice vinegar

- ¼ cup mirin or white wine vinegar

Directions:

1. In a large saucepan, bring the water to a boil.

2. Add the quinoa to the boiling water, stir, cover, and reduce the heat to low. Simmer for 15 to 20 minutes until the liquid is absorbed. Remove from the heat and let stand for 5 minutes. Fluff with a fork. Add the vinegar and mirin, and stir to combine well.

3. Divide the quinoa evenly among 4 mason jars or single-serving containers. Let cool before sealing the lids.

Nutrition: Calories: 192 Total fat: 3g Carbohydrates: 34g Fiber: 3g

14. Steamed Cauliflower

Preparation Time: 5 minutes

Cooking Time: 10 minutes

Servings: 4

Ingredients:

- 1 large head cauliflower

- 1 cup water

- ½ teaspoon salt

- 1 teaspoon red pepper flakes (optional)

Directions:

1. Remove any leaves from the cauliflower and cut it into florets.

2. In a large saucepan, bring the water to a boil. Place a steamer basket over the water and add the florets and salt. Cover and steam for 5 to 7 minutes, until tender.

3. In a large bowl, toss the cauliflower with the red pepper flakes (if using).

4. Transfer the florets to a large airtight container or 6 single-serving containers. Let cool before sealing the lids.

Nutrition: Calories: 35 Total fat: 0g Carbohydrates: 7g Fiber: 4g

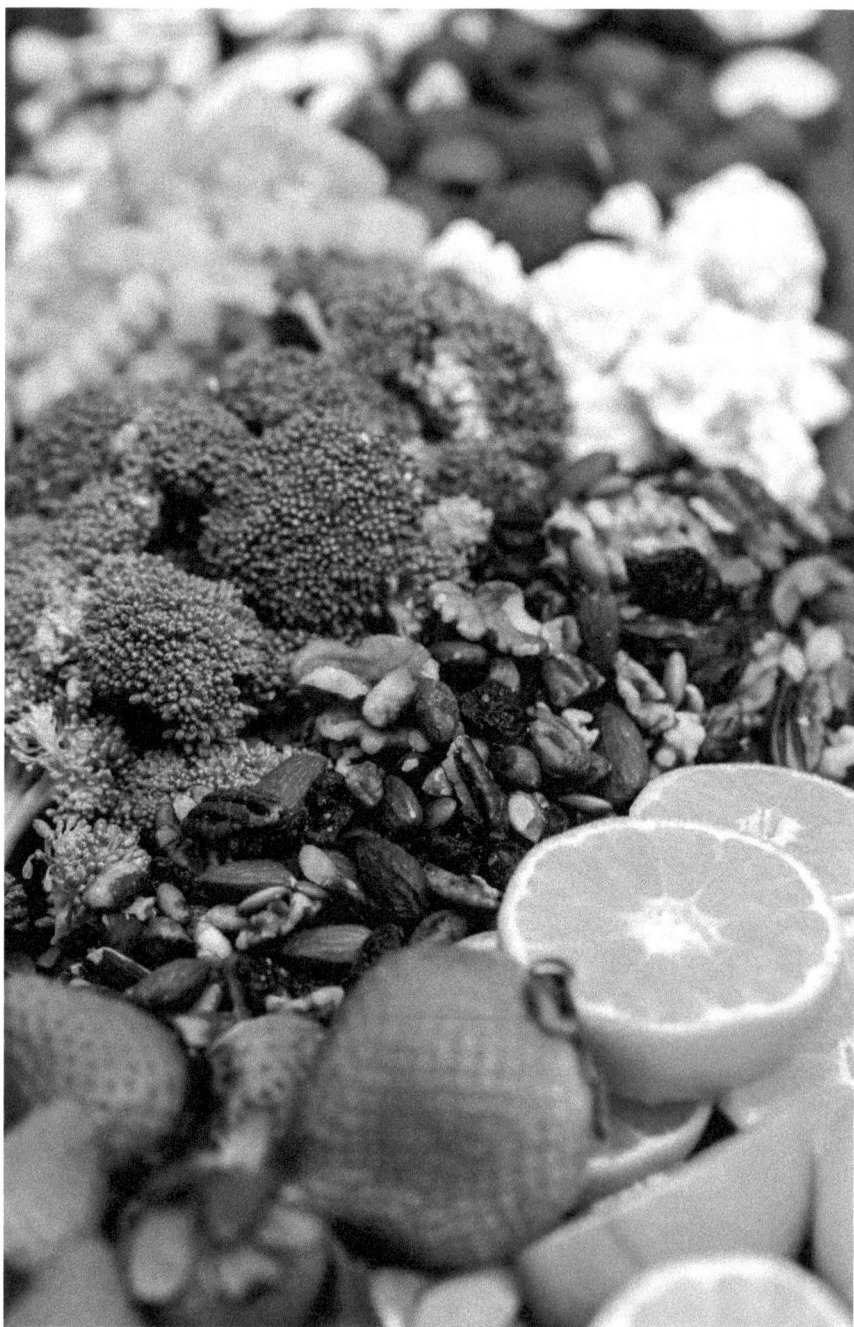

CHAPTER 3:

MAIN MEALS RECIPES

15. Mango Satay Tempeh Bowl

Preparation Time: 15 minutes

Cooking Time: 30 minutes

Servings: 4

Ingredients:

- 1 cup Black beans (cooked or canned)

- ½ cup Quinoa (dry)

- 1 14-ounces pack Tempeh (sliced)

- 1 cup Peanut butter

- 1 cup Mango cubes (frozen or fresh)

Directions:

1. Soak and cook ⅓ cup (56 g.) of dry black beans according to the method and cook the quinoa according to the package instructions.

2. Blend the mango into a smooth puree using a blender or food processor or blender and set it aside.

3. Add the tempeh slices and the peanut butter to an airtight container.

4. Close the lid and shake well until the tempeh slices are evenly covered with the peanut butter.

5. Preheat your oven and set it to 375°F. Line a baking sheet using parchment paper.

6. Transfer the peanut butter tempeh slices to the baking sheet. Bake for15 minutes or until tempeh is browned and crispy.

7. Divide the black beans, quinoa, mango puree, and tempeh slices between two bowls, serve with the optional toppings and enjoy!

Nutrition: Calories: 732 Carbs: 39 g. Fat: 42.2 g. Protein: 46.2 g

16. Fried Rice with Tofu Scramble

Preparation Time: 15 minutes

Cooking Time: 35 minutes

Servings: 2

Ingredients:

- 4 cups Quick-cooking brown rice (cooked)

- 1 cup Green peas and Carrots (julienned)

- 1 7-oz pack Extra-firm tofu (scrambled)

- ¼ cup Curry spices

- 1 cup Water

Directions:

1. Cook brown rice according to the instructions.

2. Put the pan over medium heat and add ½ cup of water and the tofu scramble.

3. Add the curry spices and cook for about 5 minutes, stirring occasionally to prevent the tofu from sticking to the pan, until the tofu is well heated and most of the water has evaporated.

4. Add the carrots, rice, and green peas along with the remaining ½ cup water and stir-fry until the water evaporated.

5. Turn off the heat, divide the fried rice between 2 bowls, serve with the optional toppings, and enjoy!

Nutrition: Calories: 285 Carbs: 30.2 g. Fat: 10.2 g. Protein: 18.1 g.

17. <u>Soy Mince Noodle Bowl</u>

Preparation Time: 15 minutes

Cooking Time: 15 minutes

Servings: 2

Ingredients:

- 2 packs Brown rice noodles

- 1 7-ounces pack textured soy mince

- 2 yellow onions (minced)

- 4 cloves Garlic (minced)

- ¼ cup Low-sodium soy sauce

- 1½ cups Water

Directions:

1. Cook noodles according to the instructions, then drain the excess water with a strainer and set aside.

2. Put a pot and turn it in a medium heat. Add ½ cup of water, the soy sauce, minced onion, and garlic.

3. Add the soy mince and cook for about 5 minutes, stirring occasionally to prevent the soy mince from sticking to the pan, until the mince has cooked and half of the water has evaporated.

4. Add the remaining water, then bring to boil while stirring occasionally.

5. Turn off the heat, add the noodles, and stir well until everything is evenly mixed.

6. Divide the noodles and mince between 2 bowls, serve with the optional toppings, and enjoy!

Nutrition: Calories: 226 Carbs: 26.3 g. Fat: 0.7 g. Protein: 25.3 g.

CHAPTER 4:

VEGETABLES, SALADS AND

SIDES RECIPES

18. Potato & Cauliflower Mash

Preparation Time: 5 minutes

Cooking Time: 25 minutes

Servings: 8

Ingredients:

- 3 cups water

- 4 lbs. potatoes (peeled)

- 16 oz. cauliflower florets

- 1 teaspoon coarse rock salt

- 2 tablespoons full cream

- Additional salt and pepper to taste

Directions:

1. Add water, potatoes, cauliflower, and salt to the Instant Pot.

2. Make sure that the lid is closed tightly and select the "Manual" function for 25 minutes with high pressure.

3. After the beep, do a Natural release in 10 minutes and remove the lid.

4. Drain the water from the pot and leave the potatoes and cauliflower inside.

5. Use a potato masher to mash the cauliflower and potatoes in the pot.

6. Stir in cream, pepper, and additional salt and mix them well.

7. Serve and enjoy.

Nutrition: Calories: 204 Carbohydrate: 38.7g Protein: 6.6g Fat: 2.1g

19. <u>Green Beans Salad</u>

Preparation Time: 5 minutes

Cooking Time: 7 minutes

Servings: 4

Ingredients:

- ½ oz. dry porcini mushrooms, soaked

- 1 cup water

- 1 lb. green beans, trimmed

- 1 lb. potatoes, quartered

- ½ teaspoon sea salt, divided

- Ground black pepper to taste

Directions:

1. Add water, potatoes, mushrooms, and salt to the Instant Pot.

2. Place the steamer trivet over the potatoes. Arrange all the green beans in the steamer.

3. Make sure that the lid is closed tightly and select the "Manual" function for 7 minutes with high pressure.

4. After the beep, do a Natural release in 10 minutes and remove the lid.

5. Transfer the greens to a platter. Strain the potatoes and mushrooms.

6. Add the potatoes and mushroom to the green beans.

7. Mix gently, sprinkle some pepper and salt on top, and serve.

Nutrition: Calories: 127 Carbohydrate: 27.7g Protein: 4.9g Fat: 0.3g

20. Instant Mashed Potato

Preparation Time: 5 minutes

Cooking Time: 18 minutes

Servings: 4

Ingredients:

- 2 cups water

- 6-8 medium potatoes (peeled)

- 1 teaspoon coarse rock salt

- 2 tablespoons full cream

- Additional salt and pepper to taste

Directions:

1. Put some water, potatoes, and salt in the Instant Pot.

2. Make sure that the lid is closed tightly and select the "Manual" function for 18 minutes with high pressure.

3. After the beep, do a Natural release in 10 minutes and remove the lid.

4. Drain the water from the pot and leave the potatoes inside.

5. To smash the potato in the pot use a masher equipment.

6. Stir in cream, pepper, and additional salt and mix them well.

7. Enjoy

Nutrition: Calories: 394 Carbohydrate: 62.5g Protein: 10.3g Fat: 9.9g

21. Cheesy Jacket Potato

Preparation Time: 10 minutes

Cooking Time: 20 minutes

Servings: 5

Ingredients:

- 5 medium potatoes

- 2 cups water

- 1 ½ tablespoons butter

- Salt and Pepper to taste

- ¼ cup cheddar cheese, shredded

- ¼ cup mozzarella cheese, shredded

- 1 teaspoon red pepper flakes

Directions:

1. Prick all the potatoes in the center and create a slit on top.

2. Top the potatoes with cheeses, butter, salt, pepper, and pepper flakes.

3. Add water to the Instant Pot and place a steamer trivet inside.

4. Arrange stuffed potatoes over the trivet with their pricked side up.

5. Secure the lid and cook on the "Manual" function for 20 minutes at high pressure.

6. When the timer goes off, do a 'Natural release' and remove the lid.

7. Transfer the potatoes to the platter and sprinkle with some salt and pepper.

8. Serve and enjoy.

Nutrition: Calories: 205 Carbohydrate: 33.8g Protein: 5.5g Fat: 5.9g

22. <u>Green Beans with Tomatoes</u>

Preparation Time: 5 minutes

Cooking Time: 7 minutes

Servings: 8

Ingredients:

- 2 tablespoons olive oil

- 2 garlic cloves, crushed

- 4 cups fresh tomatoes, diced

- 2 lbs. green beans

- Salt to taste

Directions:

1. Add oil and garlic to the Instant Pot and "Sauté" for 1 minute.

2. Stir in tomatoes and sauté for another minute.

3. Set the steamer trivet in the pot and arrange green beans over it.

4. Secure the lid and select the "Manual" function with high pressure for 5 minutes.

5. After it is done, do a Natural release to release the steam.

6. Remove the lid and the trivet along with green beans.

7. Add the beans to the tomatoes in the pot.

8. Sprinkle salt and stir well. Serve hot.

Nutrition: Calories: 82 Carbohydrate: 11.8g Protein: 2.9g Fat: 3.8g

23. <u>Wine-glazed Mushrooms</u>

Preparation Time: 5 minutes

Cooking Time: 6 minutes

Servings: 6

Ingredients:

- 2 tablespoons olive oil

- 6 garlic cloves, minced

- 2 lbs. fresh mushrooms, sliced

- 1/3 cup balsamic vinegar

- 1/3 cup white wine

- Salt and black pepper to taste

Directions:

1. Put some oil and garlic in the Instant Pot and Select the "Sauté" function to cook for 1 minute.

2. Now add all the remaining ingredients to the cooker.

3. Switch the cooker to the "Manual" function with high pressure and 5 minutes cooking time.

4. After it is done, do a Quick release, then remove the lid?

5. Sprinkle some salt and black pepper if desired, then serve.

Nutrition: Calories: 91 Carbohydrate: 6.5g Protein: 5g Fat: 5.1g

24. Steamed Garlic Broccoli

Preparation Time: 5 minutes

Cooking Time: 10 minutes

Servings: 6

Ingredients:

- 6 cups broccoli florets

- 1 cup water

- ½ garlic cloves, minced

- 2 tablespoons peanut oil

- 2 tablespoons Chinese rice wine

- Fine Sea Salt, to taste

- Lemon slices to garnish

Directions:

1. Put some water into the insert of Instant Pot.

2. Place the steamer trivet inside.

3. Arrange the broccoli florets over the trivet.

4. Make sure that the lid is close tightly and select the "Manual" function with low pressure for 5 minutes.

5. After the beep, do a Natural release and remove the lid.

6. Strain the florets and return them back to the pot. Add the remaining ingredients to the broccoli.

7. Select "Sauté" and stir-fry for 5 minutes.

8. Garnish with lemon slices and serve.

Nutrition Calories: 72 Carbohydrate: 6.1g Protein: 2.6g Fat: 4.8g

25. Lime Potatoes

Preparation Time: 5 minutes

Cooking Time: 10 minutes

Servings: 2

Ingredients:

- ½ tablespoon olive oil

- 2 ½ medium potatoes, scrubbed and cubed

- 1 tablespoon fresh rosemary, chopped

- Freshly ground black pepper to taste

- ½ cup vegetable broth

- 1 tablespoon fresh lemon juice

Directions:

1. Put the oil, potatoes, pepper, and rosemary in the Instant Pot.

2. "Sauté" for 4 minutes with constant stirring.

3. Put all the remaining ingredients into the Instant Pot.

4. Make sure that the lid is closed tightly and select the "Manual" function for 6 minutes with high pressure.

5. Do a quick release after the beep and then remove the lid.

6. Give a gentle stir and serve warm.

Nutrition: Calories: 225 Carbohydrate: 43.3g Protein: 5.1g Fat: 4.1g

CHAPTER 5:

DESSERT RECIPES

26. Mexican Chocolate Mousse

Preparation Time: 15 minutes

Cooking Time: 0 minutes

Servings: 4

Ingredients:

- 8 ounces bittersweet or semisweet vegan chocolate

- 1¾ cups (about 1 pound) silken tofu

- ½ cup pure maple syrup

- 1 teaspoon vanilla

- 1½ teaspoons ground cinnamon

Directions:

1. Create a double boiler by bringing a medium pot filled halfway with water to a low simmer. Place a heatproof bowl above and make sure it is not touching the water. Add the chocolate to the bowl. Keep the pot over low heat and stir the chocolate until it is melted and silky smooth.

2. In a food processor, add all the ingredients. Blend until smooth.

3. Refrigerate before serving.

4. Substitution Tip: Substitute 1 teaspoon of chili powder for the ground cinnamon or add both for an authentic Mexican chocolate experience.

Nutrition: Calories: 442 Fat: 18g Carbohydrate: 68g Protein: 12g

27. Chocolate Peanut Butter Cups

Preparation Time: 20 minutes

Cooking Time: 0 minutes

Servings: 8

Ingredients:

- 5 ounces vegan semisweet chocolate, divided

- ½ cup smooth peanut butter

- ½ teaspoon vanilla

- ¼ teaspoon salt

Directions:

1. Line a muffin tray with 9 mini or regular paper cupcake liners.

2. Place half the chocolate in a microwave-safe bowl and microwave on high for 25 seconds, then take it out and stir.

3. Place bowl back in the microwave and repeat the process of cooking for 25 seconds, stopping and stirring, until the chocolate has melted.

4. Spoon 1 to 1½ teaspoons of melted chocolate into each cup. Place in the refrigerator for 10 minutes until solid.

5. Stir the peanut butter, vanilla, and salt together in a bowl. Transfer the peanut butter mixture to a resealable plastic bag and seal it tightly. Cut one corner of the plastic bag, then squeeze the bag to pipe 2 to 3 teaspoons of peanut butter in the middle of each cup. Smooth with a small spoon.

6. Melt the remaining chocolate. Spoon 1 to 1½ teaspoons of chocolate into the top of each cup. Smooth with a small spoon.

7. Refrigerate until solid, 30 to 40 minutes. Peel off the liners and enjoy. Remove it from the refrigerator. Let it sit for 15 or a few minutes if you like a softer chocolate.

8. Leftovers: Store leftovers in the refrigerator for up to 2 weeks or in the freezer for up to 1 month.

Nutrition: Calories: 177 Fat: 13g Carbohydrate: 15g Protein: 5g

28. Banana Ice Cream with Chocolate Sauce

Preparation Time: 10 minutes

Cooking Time: 0 minutes

Servings: 4

Ingredients:

- ½ cup raw unsalted cashews

- ¼ cup pure maple syrup

- 1 tablespoon unsweetened cocoa powder

- 1 teaspoon vanilla extract

- ¼ teaspoon salt

- ¼ cup water

- 6 ripe bananas, peeled and frozen

Directions:

1. Place cashews in a bowl and put water. Soak cashews for two hours or overnight. Drain and rinse.

2. In a food processor or blender, place the cashews, maple syrup, cocoa powder, vanilla, and salt. Blend, adding the water a couple of tablespoons at a time until you get a smooth consistency.

3. Transfer to an airtight container, then refrigerate. Bring to room temperature before using.

4. Place frozen bananas in the food processor. Process until you have smooth banana ice cream. Serve topped with chocolate sauce.

5. Ingredient Tip: The best way to freeze a banana is to start with ripe peeled bananas. Slice them into 2-inch chunks and arrange them in a single layer on a parchment-lined baking sheet. Pop them in the freezer. Once frozen, transfer to freezer-safe bags. Frozen bananas are also a delicious, healthy addition to smoothies. Individually freeze chunks of one banana, and you'll always be ready to create an icy, rich, creamy smoothie.

Nutrition: Calories: 301 Fat: 8g Carbohydrate: 59g Protein: 5g

CHAPTER 6:

SNACK RECIPES

29. Pumpkin Garam Masala

Preparation Time: 10 minutes

Cooking Time: 30 minutes

Servings: 4

Ingredients:

- 2 tablespoons olive oil

- 1 sweet onion, finely chopped

- 2 teaspoons minced garlic

- 4 cups diced fresh or frozen pumpkin

- 2 (15-ounce) cans white kidney beans, drained and rinsed

- 2 tomatoes, diced

- 1 cup low-sodium vegetable stock

- 2 tablespoons garam masala spice

Directions:

1. In a saucepan, put olive oil, then turn it in medium-high heat.

2. Sauté the onion and garlic until softened, about 3 minutes.

3. Stir in the pumpkin, beans, tomatoes, vegetable stock, and garam masala.

4. Bring the curry to boil and then reduce the heat to low and simmer until the pumpkin is tender, about 25 minutes.

Nutrition: Calories: 235 Total Fat: 8g Protein: 12g Cholesterol: 0mg Sodium: 17mg Carbohydrates: 33g Fiber: 8g

30. Spicy Tomato Braised Chickpeas

Preparation Time: 10 minutes

Cooking Time: 20 minutes

Servings: 4

Ingredients:

- 1 tablespoon olive oil

- 1 sweet onion, finely chopped

- 1 tablespoon minced garlic

- 2 (15-ounce) cans crushed tomatoes

- 2 (15-ounce) cans chickpeas, drained and rinsed

- ½ cup finely chopped fresh basil

- ⅛ Teaspoon red pepper flakes

- Sea salt, for seasoning

- Freshly ground black pepper, for seasoning

- 3 zucchini, spiralized

Directions:

1. Prepare, then heat the olive oil in a saucepan in medium-high heat.

2. Sauté the onion and garlic until softened, about 3 minutes.

3. Stir in the tomatoes, chickpeas, basil, and red pepper flakes.

4. Reduce to low heat if the sauce is already boiling, then simmer for 10 minutes to reduce the liquid slightly.

5. Season the sauce with salt and pepper.

6. Serve over spiralized zucchini.

Nutrition: Calories: 415 Total Fat: 6g Protein: 18g Cholesterol: 0mg Sodium: 215mg Carbohydrates: 74g Fiber: 18g

31. Baked Zucchini Chips

Preparation Time: 10 minutes

Cooking Time: 2 hours and 45 minutes

Servings: 10

Ingredients:

- 2 medium zucchini, sliced with a mandolin

- 1 tablespoon olive oil

- 1/2 teaspoon salt

Directions:

1. Preheat your oven to 200 degrees F.

2. Prepare a parchment paper and line it with the baking sheets.

3. Mix every ingredient in the large bowl and toss to thoroughly coat the zucchini with oil and salt.

4. Single later the zucchini slices on the baking sheet. It should not overlap.

5. Bake it in the oven for 2 and a half hours or until the zucchini chips are golden and crispy.

6. Turn the off oven, then allow it to cool with the oven door slightly open. This will allow the zucchini chips to crisp up even more as they cool.

Nutrition: Fat: 1.5g Carbohydrates: 1.3g Protein: 0.5g

32. Ice-cream

Preparation Time: 10 minutes

Cooking Time: 1 hour 10 minutes

Servings: 6

Ingredients:

- 1 ½ cup full fat coconut milk

- ⅓ Cup natural peanut butter

- 2 tablespoons vanilla extract

- ⅛ Teaspoon stevia powder

- A pinch of salt

Directions:

1. Prior to starting this recipe, place a freezer-safe container in the freezer for at least 24 hours before to ensure that when the ice cream mixture is transferred no ice crystals are formed.

2. Blend all the ingredients and blend until a smooth and creamy consistency is achieved.

3. Chill this mixture by placing it in the refrigerator for 1 hour.

4. Transfer the mixture to an ice-cream maker and churn for 10 minutes or until it achieves a soft serve consistency.

5. Transfer the ice cream to the prepared freezer-safe container and freeze for at least one hour before serving. Can be served with caramel sauce.

Nutrition: Fat: 10.1g Carbohydrates: 3.7 Protein: 4.7g

33. Peanut Butter Cups

Preparation Time: 10 minutes

Cooking Time: 45 minutes

Servings: 18

Ingredients:

- ½ cup peanut butter

- 1 cup sugar-free dark chocolate chips

- 1 tablespoon coconut oil

Directions:

1. Get a microwave-safe bowl and place all the chocolate chips and coconut oil in the bowl. Microwave in 15 second bursts to melt the chocolate. Stir to combine the two ingredients.

2. Put a spoonful of chocolate into foil candy cups. Swirl so that the chocolate coats the sides of the cups. Pour excess chocolate back into the bowl.

3. Place the chocolate lined cups in the freezer for 10 minutes or until chocolate is set.

4. While the chocolate is setting, place the peanut butter in a microwave-safe bowl and microwave in 15 second bursts until the peanut butter becomes pourable.

5. Pour a spoonful of peanut butter into each of the chocolate-set cups. Make sure that the cup is a flat surface to smooth the tops of the peanut butter.

6. Pour a tablespoon of melted chocolate on top of the peanut butter in each cup.

7. Place it in the freezer for about 10 minutes to set chocolate. Unmold and serve. This can be stored using an airtight container and refrigerate for up to 3 days, or you can make it last in the freezer for a month.

8. Put it in the freezer for at least 10 minutes to set the chocolate. Then serve. Using an airtight container, you can refrigerate it for up to 3 days.

Nutrition: Fat: 5.7g Carbohydrates: 3.2g Protein: 2g

34. Quick Peanut Butter Bars

Preparation Time: 10 minutes

Cooking Time: 0 minutes

Servings: 10

Ingredients:

- 20 soft-pitted Medjool dates

- 1 cup of raw almonds

- 1 ¼ cup of crushed pretzels

- 1/3 cup of natural peanut butter

Directions:

1. Transfer your almonds to a food processor and mix them until they are broken.

2. Add the peanut butter and the dates. Blend them until you have a thick dough

3. Crush the pretzels and put them in the processor. Pulse enough to mix them with the rest of the ingredients. You can also give them a good stir with a spoon.

4. Take a small, square pan and line it with parchment paper. Press the dough onto the pan, flattening it with your hands or a spoon.

5. Put it in the freezer for about 2 hours or in the fridge for about 4 hours.

6. Once it is fully set, cut it into bars. Store them and enjoy them when you are hungry. Just remember to store them in a sealed container.

Nutrition: Calories: 343 Fat 23 g Carbohydrates 33 g Protein 5 g

35. Hummus without Oil

Preparation Time: 5 minutes

Cooking Time: 0 minutes

Servings: 6

Ingredients:

- 2 tablespoons of lemon juice

- 1 15-ounce can of chickpeas

- 2 tablespoons of tahini

- 1-2 freshly chopped/minced garlic cloves

- Red pepper hummus

- 2 tablespoons of almond milk pepper

Directions:

1. Wash with running water the chickpeas and put them in a high-speed blender with garlic. Blend them until they break into fine pieces.

2. Add the other ingredients and blend everything until you have a smooth paste. Add some water if you want a less thick consistency.

3. Your homemade hummus dip is ready to be served with eatables

Nutrition: Calories: 202 Fat 3 g Carbohydrates 35 g Protein 11 g

36. Spiced Kale Chips

Preparation Time: 10 minutes

Cooking Time: 30 minutes

Servings: 4

Ingredients:

- 1 bunch curly kale

- 1 tablespoon olive oil

- ¼ teaspoon of salt

- ⅛ Teaspoon garlic powder

- ⅛ Teaspoon black pepper

Directions:

1. Preheat the oven to 300 degrees F.

2. Prepare an aluminum foil and line it in a baking sheet pan.

3. Rinse and dry kale thoroughly by spinning in a salad spinner or patting it with paper towels.

4. Tear kale leaves off the stems and break into pieces the size of potato chips. Place into a large mixing bowl and add the rest of

the ingredients. Toss so that the kale leaves are thoroughly coated with the spices and oil.

5. Place the coated kale leaves in an even layer that does not overlap on a wire baking rack. Place the wire baking rack atop the foil lined baking sheet.

6. Bake it for 20 minutes or wait until the kale leaves are crispy.

7. Allow to cool and serve.

Nutrition: Fat: 3g Carbohydrates: 1.8g Protein: 0.9g

37. Coconut Fat Cups

Preparation Time: 10 minutes

Cooking Time: 15 minutes

Servings: 10

Ingredients:

- ¼ cup coconut butter, melted

- ¼ cup coconut oil, melted

- 3 drops liquid stevia

- ⅓ Cup shredded coconut

Directions:

1. Mix the ingredients in a medium bowl and thoroughly combine.

2. Using a tablespoon, fill mini cupcake liners or an ice cube tray with the mixture.

3. Freeze for at least 1 hour and serve. Using an airtight container, you can refrigerate it for up until 2 days.

Nutrition: Fat: 11.7g Carbohydrates: 2.5g Protein: 0.7g

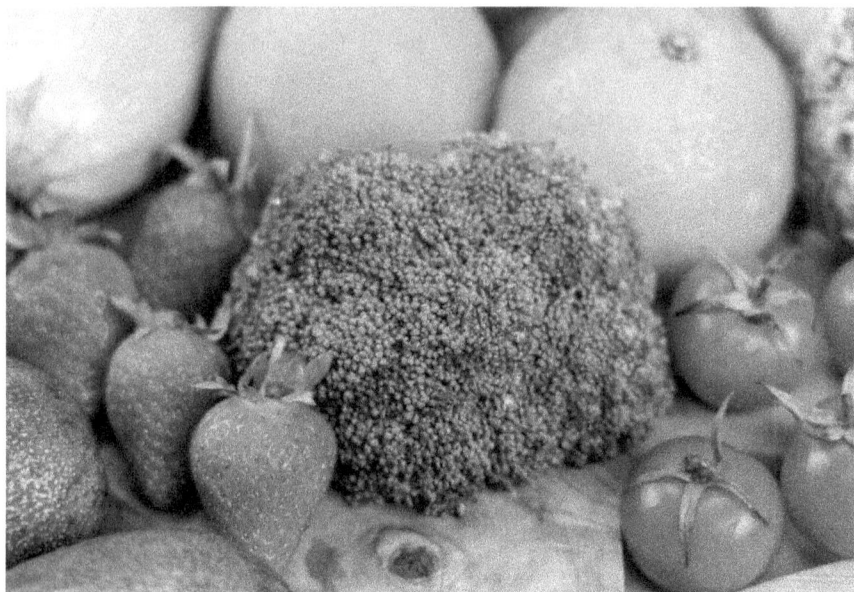

CHAPTER 7:

JUICES AND SMOOTHIES

RECIPES

38. Pineapple Smoothie

Preparation Time: 5 minutes Cooking Time: 0 minutes

Servings: 2

Ingredients:

- ½ cup of fresh pineapple

- ½ cup of strawberry

- 1 banana

- ¼ cup of orange juice

- Mint ice cubes

Directions:

1. Place the pineapple juice, banana, frozen pineapple, and vanilla Greek yogurt in a blender.

2. Blend until smooth.

3. Pour into 2 glasses. Garnish with pineapple wedges and mint sprigs if desired.

Calories: 169 Carbohydrates: 33g Protein: 6g Cholesterol: 2mg Sodium: 33mg Fiber: 7g Sugar: 35g

39. Sweet Smoothie

Preparation Time: 5 minutes

Cooking Time: 0 minutes

Servings: 2

Ingredients:

- 1 banana

- 1 sliced mango

- 1 cup fresh pineapple

- 1 tablespoon peanut butter

- ½ coconut water

Directions:

1. Process the banana, mango, pineapple, peanut butter, and coconut water in a blender until smooth and creamy.

2. Enjoy immediately or keep cool in the refrigerator.

Nutrition: Calories: 168 Fat: 0.7g Carbohydrates: 42.3g Protein: 1.5g Cholesterol: 0mg Sodium: 5mg

40. Strawberry-Flax Smoothie

Preparation Time: 5 minutes

Cooking Time: 0 minutes

Servings: 1

Ingredients:

- 1 cup of frozen strawberries

- ¾ cup plain low-fat yogurt

- ½ cup fresh orange juice

- 1 tablespoon honey

- 1 tablespoon flaxseed meal

Directions:

1. Combine the strawberries, yogurt, orange juice, honey, and flaxseed meal in a blender.

2. Blend until smooth.

Nutrition: Calories: 334 Fat: 7g Cholesterol: 11mg, Sodium: 134mg Protein: 14g Carbohydrate: 58g Sugar: 49g Fiber: 6g

41. <u>Coconut Milk Smoothie</u>

Preparation Time: 5 minutes

Cooking Time: 0 minutes

Servings: 4

Ingredients:

- 1 10-ounce frozen blueberries

- 1 cup plain yogurt

- 3 ripe bananas

- 1 cup unsweetened coconut milk

- 2 tablespoons honey

Directions:

1. Combine the blueberries, bananas, yogurt, coconut milk, and honey in a blender and serve.

Nutrition: Calories: 300 Fat: 15g Cholesterol: 10mg Sodium: 40mg Carbohydrate: 43g Fiber: 3g Sugar: 28g Protein: 5g

42. Spiced Pumpkin Smoothie

Preparation Time: 5 minutes

Cooking Time: 0 minutes

Servings: 1

Ingredients:

- 1 cup ice

- ½ cup whole milk

- ⅓ Cup pure pumpkin puree

- 1 tablespoon honey

- Pinch of ground nutmeg

Directions:

1. Place the ice, milk, pumpkin puree, honey, and nutmeg in a blender.

2. Blend until smooth.

Nutrition: Calories: 165 Fat: 4g Cholesterol: 12mg Sodium: 53mg Protein: 5g Carbohydrate: 29g Sugar: 26g Fiber: 3g

43. <u>Carrot-Pineapple Smoothie</u>

Preparation Time: 5 minutes

Cooking Time: 0 minutes

Servings: 2

Ingredients:

- ¾ cup chopped fresh pineapple

- ½ cup ice

- ⅓ Cup fresh orange juice

- ¼ cup chopped carrot

- ½ banana

Directions:

1. Place the pineapple, ice, orange juice, carrot, and banana in a blender.

2. Blend until smooth.

Nutrition: Calories: 159 Fat: 1g Cholesterol: 0mg Sodium: 25mg Protein: 2g Carbohydrate: 40g Sugar: 26g Fiber: 4g

CHAPTER 8:

OTHER RECIPES

44. Tangy Spiced Cranberry Drink

Preparation Time: 10 Minutes

Cooking Time: 2 hours and 10 minutes

Servings: 14

Ingredients:

- 1 1/2 cups of coconut sugar

- 12 whole cloves

- 2 fluid ounce of lemon juice

- 6 fluid ounce of orange juice

- 32 fluid ounce of cranberry juice

- 8 cups of hot water

- 1/2 cup of Red Hot candies

Directions:

1. Pour the water into a 6-quarts slow cooker along with the cranberry juice, orange juice, and lemon juice.

2. Stir the sugar properly.

3. Wrap the whole cloves in a cheesecloth, tie its corners with strings, and immerse it in the liquid present inside the slow cooker.

4. Add the red hot candies to the slow cooker and cover it with the lid.

5. Then plug in the slow cooker and let it cook on the low heat setting for 3 hours or until it is heated thoroughly.

6. When done, discard the cheesecloth bag and serve.

Nutrition: Calories: 89 Carbohydrates: 27g Protein: 0g Fats: 0g

45. <u>Warm Pomegranate Punch</u>

Preparation Time: 10 Minutes

Cooking Time: 2 hours and 10 minutes

Servings: 8

Ingredients:

- 3 cinnamon sticks, each about 3 inches long

- 12 whole cloves

- 1/2 cup of coconut sugar

- 1/3 cup of lemon juice

- 32 fluid ounce of pomegranate juice

- 32 fluid ounce of apple juice, unsweetened

- 16 fluid ounce of brewed tea

Directions:

1. Using a 4-quart slow cooker, pour the lemon juice, pomegranate, juice apple juice, tea, and then sugar.

2. Wrap the whole cloves and cinnamon stick in a cheesecloth, tie its corners with a string, and immerse it in the liquid present in the slow cooker.

3. Then cover it with the lid, plug in the slow cooker and let it cook at the low heat setting for 3 hours or until it is heated thoroughly.

4. When done, discard the cheesecloth bag and serve it hot or cold.

Nutrition: Calories: 253 Carbohydrates: 58g Protein: 7g Fats: 2g

46. Rich Truffle Hot Chocolate

Preparation Time: 10 Minutes

Cooking Time: 1 hour and 10 minutes

Servings: 4

Ingredients:

- 1/3 cup of cocoa powder, unsweetened

- 1/3 cup of coconut sugar

- 1/8 teaspoon of salt

- 1/8 teaspoon of ground cinnamon

- 1 teaspoon of vanilla extract, unsweetened

- 32 fluid ounce of coconut milk

Directions:

1. Using a 2 quarts slow cooker, add all the ingredients, and stir properly.

2. Cover it with the lid, then plug in the slow cooker and cook it for 2 hours on the high heat setting or until it is heated thoroughly.

3. When done, serve right away.

Nutrition: Calories: 67 Carbohydrates: 13 Protein: 2g Fats: 2g

47. Dehydrated Walnuts

Preparation Time: 15 Minutes Cooking Time: 24 Hours

Servings: 4

Ingredients:

- 1 cup walnuts, soaked overnight and drained

- 2 tablespoons dates, pitted and mashed into a paste form

- 1/8 teaspoon ground cinnamon

- Pinch of cayenne pepper

- Sea salt, as required

Directions:

1. Set the dehydrator to 100 degrees F.

2. In a large bowl, mix together all ingredients.

3. Arrange the walnuts onto the dehydrator sheets.

4. Dehydrate for about 24 hours.

5. Remove from the dehydrator and set aside to cool completely before serving.

Nutrition: Calories: 209 Fats: 18.5g Carbs: 7.4g Proteins: 7.7g

48. <u>Kale Chips</u>

Preparation Time: 10 Minutes

Cooking Time: 15 minutes

Servings: 6

Ingredients:

- 1 pound fresh kale leaves, stemmed and torn

- ¼ teaspoon cayenne pepper

- Salt, as required

- 1 tablespoon olive oil

Directions:

1. Preheat the oven to 350 degrees F. Line a large baking sheet with a parchment paper.

2. Arrange the kale pieces onto the prepared baking sheet in a single layer.

3. Sprinkle the kale with the cayenne pepper and salt and drizzle with oil.

4. Bake for about 10-15 minutes.

5. Remove from the oven and set aside to cool before serving.

Nutrition: Calories: 57 Fats: 2.3g Carbs: 8g Proteins: 2.3g

49. Beet Chips

Preparation Time: 15 Minutes

Cooking Time: 30 minutes

Servings: 4

Ingredients:

- 2 medium beets, trimmed, peeled, and sliced thinly

- 1 tablespoon canola oil

- Salt, as required

Directions:

1. Preheat the oven to 350 degrees F. Line 2 large baking sheets with parchment paper.

2. In a large bowl, add the beet slices and oil and toss to coat well.

3. Arrange the beet slices onto the prepared baking sheets in a single layer.

4. Bake for about 20-30 minutes.

5. Remove from the oven and set aside to cool before serving.

Nutrition: Calories: 53 Fats: 3.6g Carbs: 5g Proteins: 0.8g

50. Zucchini Chips

Preparation Time: 15 Minutes Cooking Time: 15 minutes

Servings: 2

Ingredients:

- 1 medium zucchini, cut into thin slices

- 1/8 teaspoon ground turmeric

- 1/8 teaspoon ground cumin

- Salt, as required

- 2 teaspoons olive oil

Directions:

1. Preheat the oven to 400 degrees F. Line 2 baking sheets with parchment papers. In a large bowl, add all ingredients and toss to coat well.

2. Transfer the mixture onto the prepared baking sheets in a single layer. Bake for about 10-15 minutes.

3. Serve immediately.

Nutrition: Calories: 57 Fats: 4.9g Carbs: 3.4g Proteins: 1.2g

CONCLUSION

Well done! Thank you for reaching the end of this book, The Complete Vegetarian Cookbook.

Hopefully, this book has helped you understand that making vegetarian recipes and diet easier can improve your life, not only by improving your health and helping you lose weight, but also by saving you money and time.

Remember that vegetarianism is a choice, not a religion.

Be flexible when it comes to your diet and enjoy new tastes and experiences.

Don't be afraid of meat substitutes, but experiment with using them sparingly. There is no need to completely replace meat with fake meat products like tofu or processed soy-based vegetarian burgers and hot dogs. Not only are they expensive, but fake meats contain artificial ingredients that may or may not be healthy for you.

Also, if you are not used to eating a vegetarian diet, start with a few vegetarian meals and snacks during the week, and see how you feel.

You can always add more vegetarian meals to your diet later. It is better to be even slightly vegetarians than completely non-vegetarian.

The best tip I can give you about making vegetarian recipes is to experiment and have fun!

Here are some more tips to help you with your vegetarian diet:

1. Remember that vegetarianism is not a destination, it is a journey.

2. A vegetarian diet is plant-based. This means that you should try to eat more plants and less animal products. You should also be careful not to replace whole foods with their processed counterparts, such as replacing whole foods such as fruits and vegetables with fruit juice and pasta sauce.

3. Try to avoid processed food whenever possible, while still maintaining your balanced diet and nutrients that you need for your health. An easier way of doing this will be to make your own food when possible and try to avoid packaged, pre-prepared foods at the grocery store.

4. Avoid processed food products that contain artificial ingredients, such as sweeteners, colors, and flavors.

5. Avoid highly processed meat substitutes. Remember to use meat substitutes in moderation or as an occasional treat.

6. If you choose to eat meat substitutes such as tofu, be sure to thoroughly cook it and try different ways of preparing it

7. You may need to gradually introduce your family and friends to your new eating habits. Don't expect everyone to support you or enjoy the same things you do when it comes to vegetarian recipes. As long as you are happy with your food choices, that is the most important thing – even if it means making some changes at home!

When you are having a hard time, always remember this: You can always choose to stop being a vegetarian.

You can simply start eating meat again if you are struggling with your new diet.

Remember that it is okay to be a part-time vegetarian, but if you find that you cannot maintain the lifestyle or are unhappy with your choice, it is always better to go back to eating a non-veg diet.

There is no shame in making changes to your vegetarian recipe routine if you need to, and you will not shame yourself for deciding that a strict vegetarian diet does not work for you.

I know that there are many books and choosing my book is amazing. I am thankful that you stopped and took the time to decide. You made a great decision, and I am sure that you enjoyed it.

I will be even happier if you will add some comments. Feedbacks helped by growing, and they still do. They help me to choose better content and new ideas. So, maybe your feedback can trigger an idea for my next book. Thank you again for downloading this book!

I hope you enjoyed reading my book!

www.ingramcontent.com/pod-product-compliance
Lightning Source LLC
Chambersburg PA
CBHW062344300326
41947CB00012B/1204